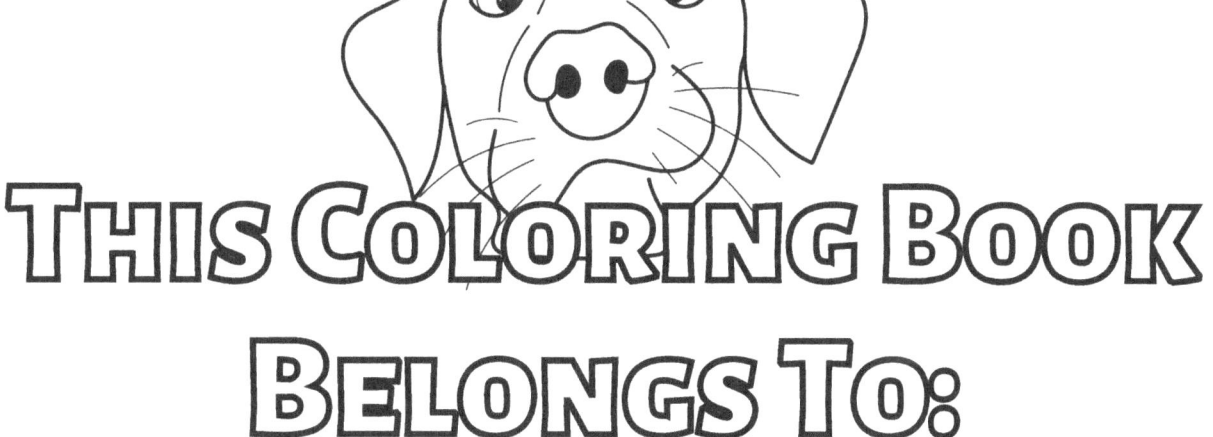

This Coloring Book Belongs To:

_____

_____

Discover More Books!

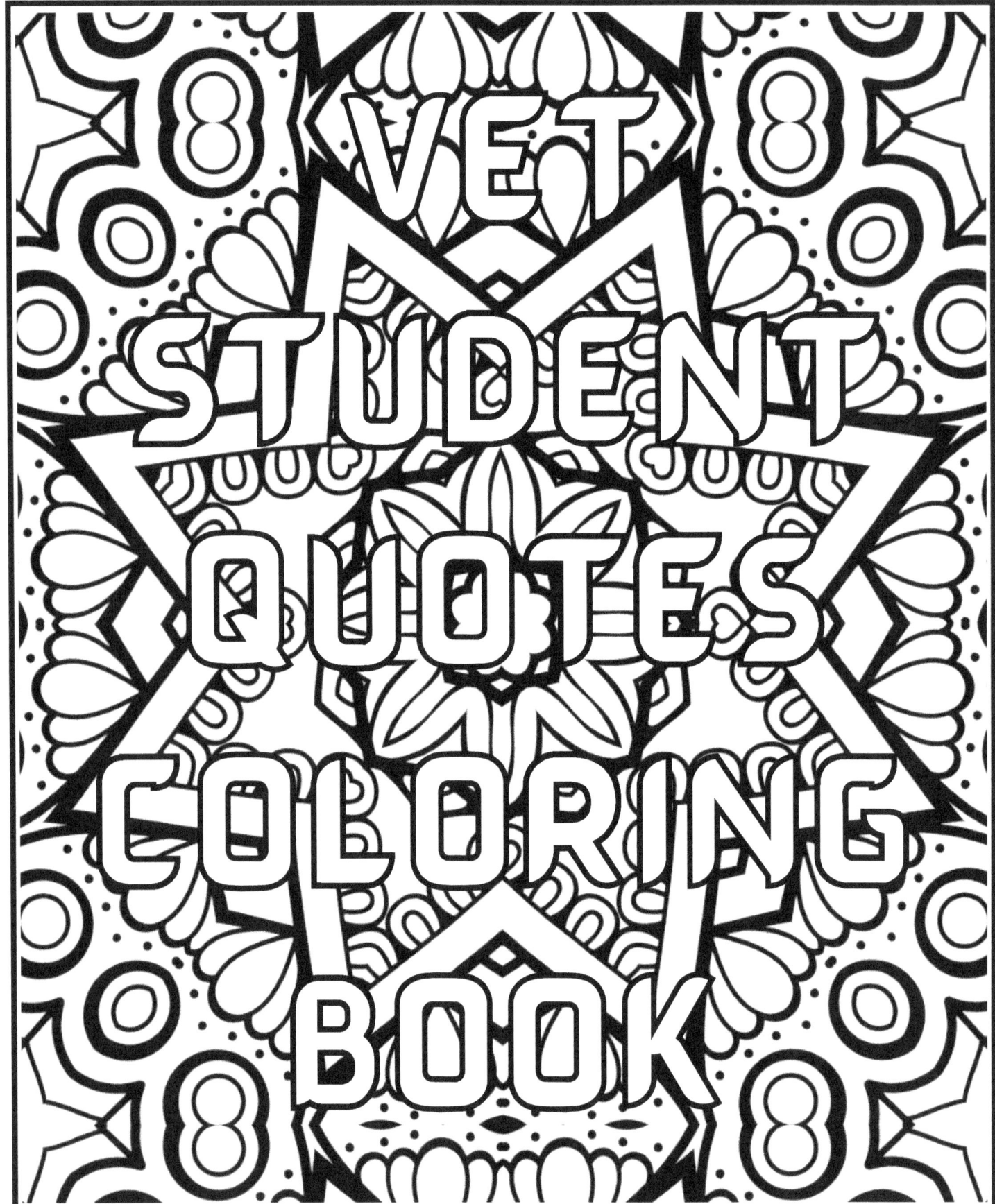

VET STUDENT QUOTES COLORING BOOK

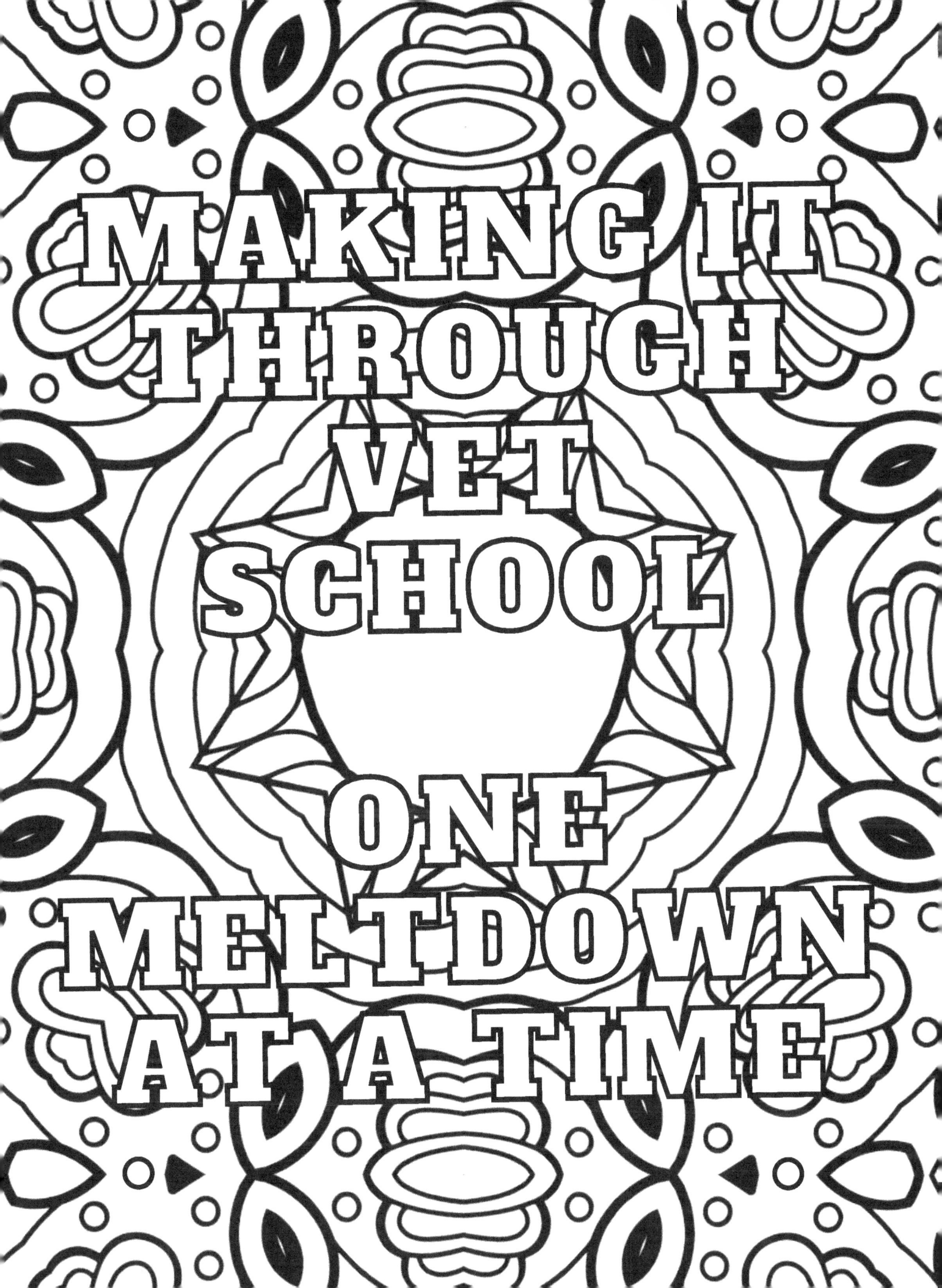

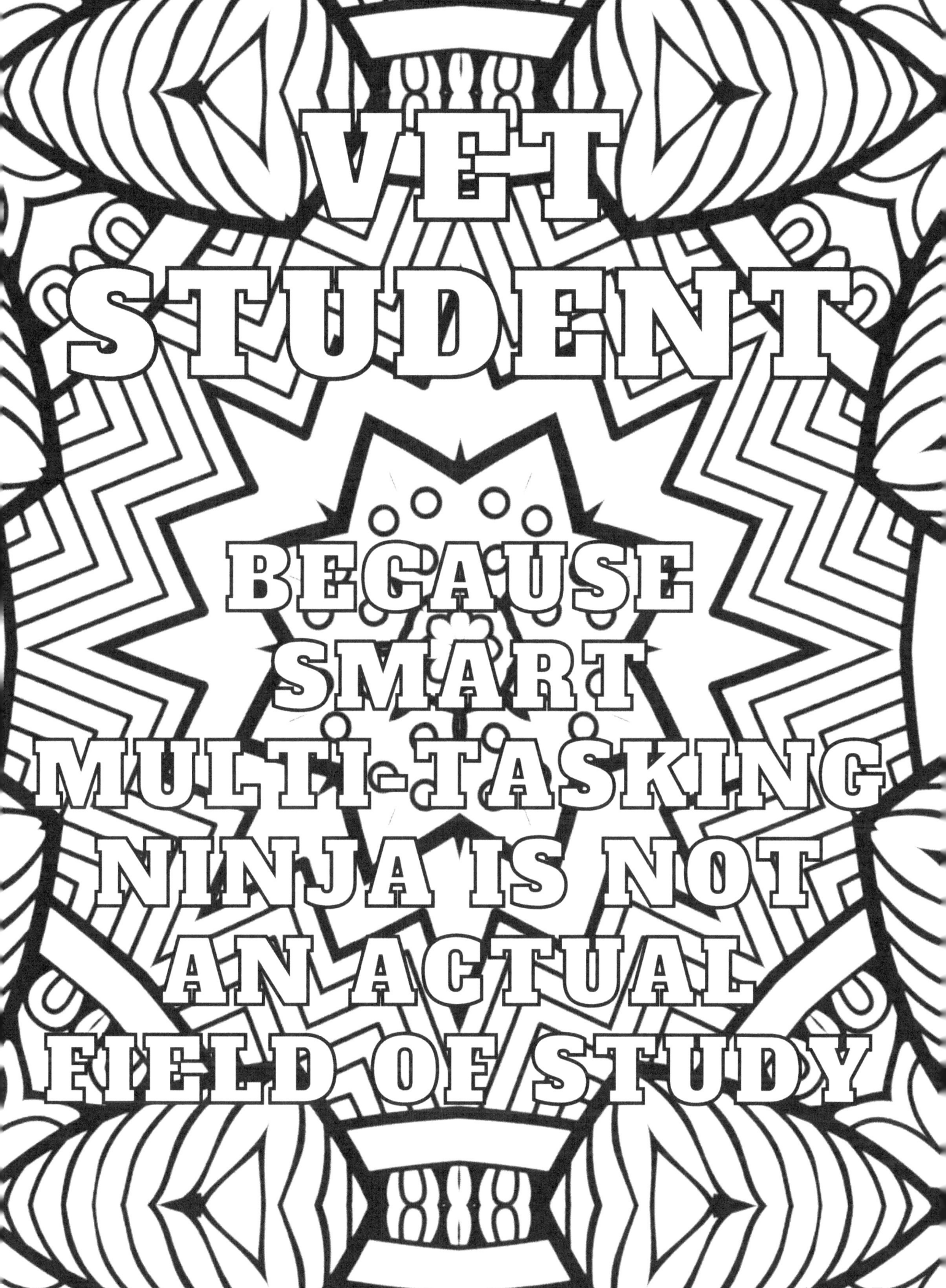

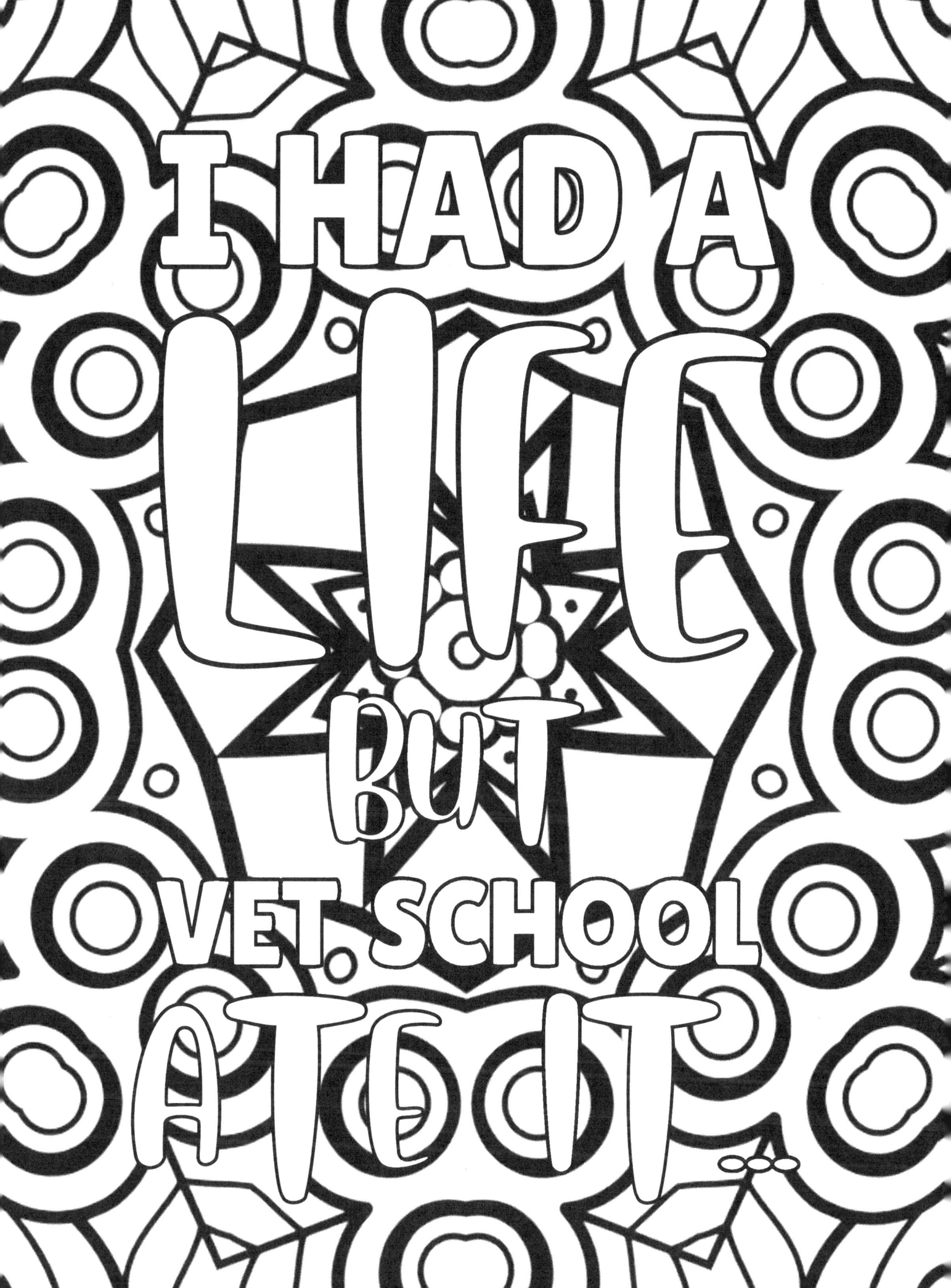

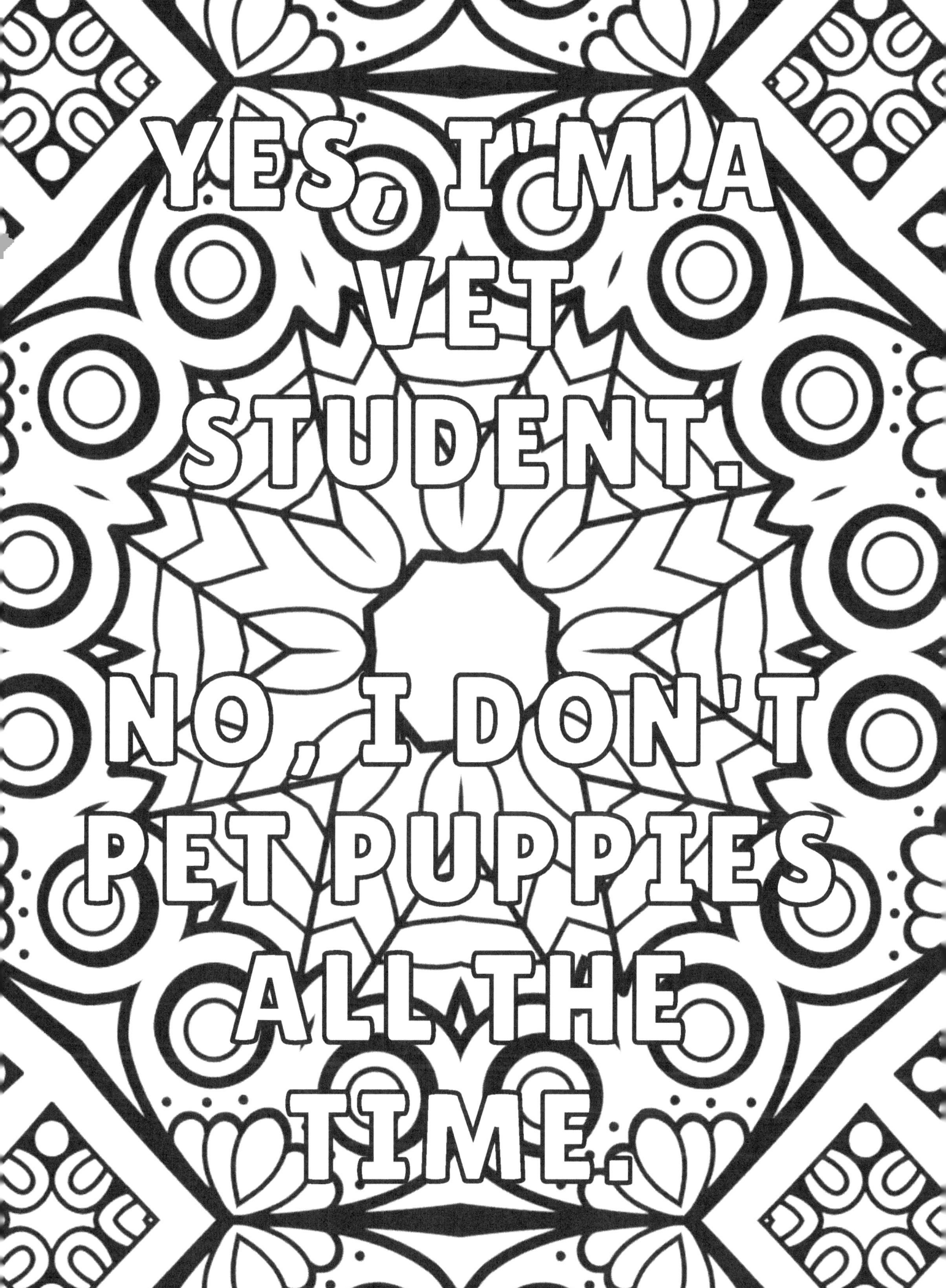

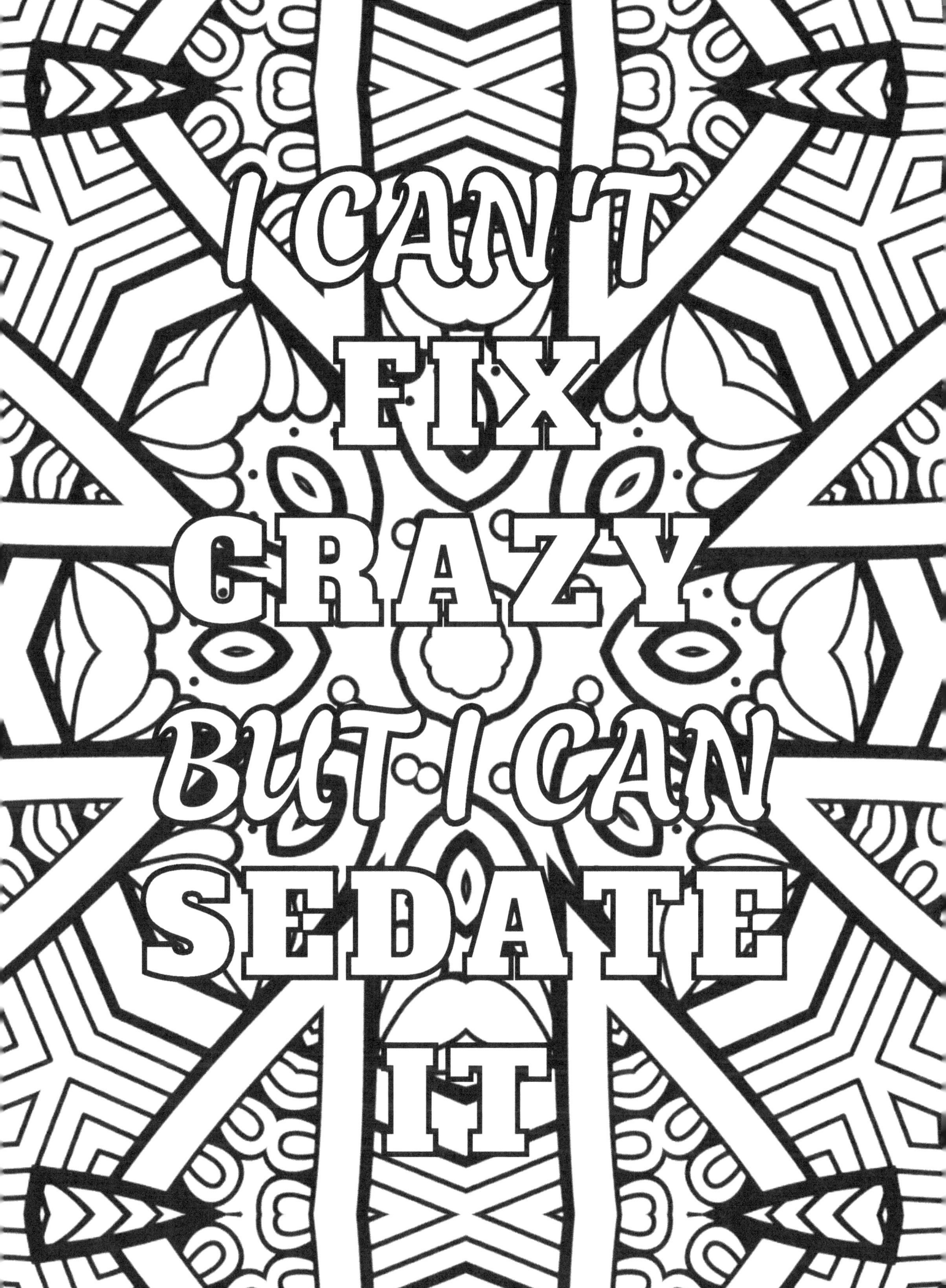

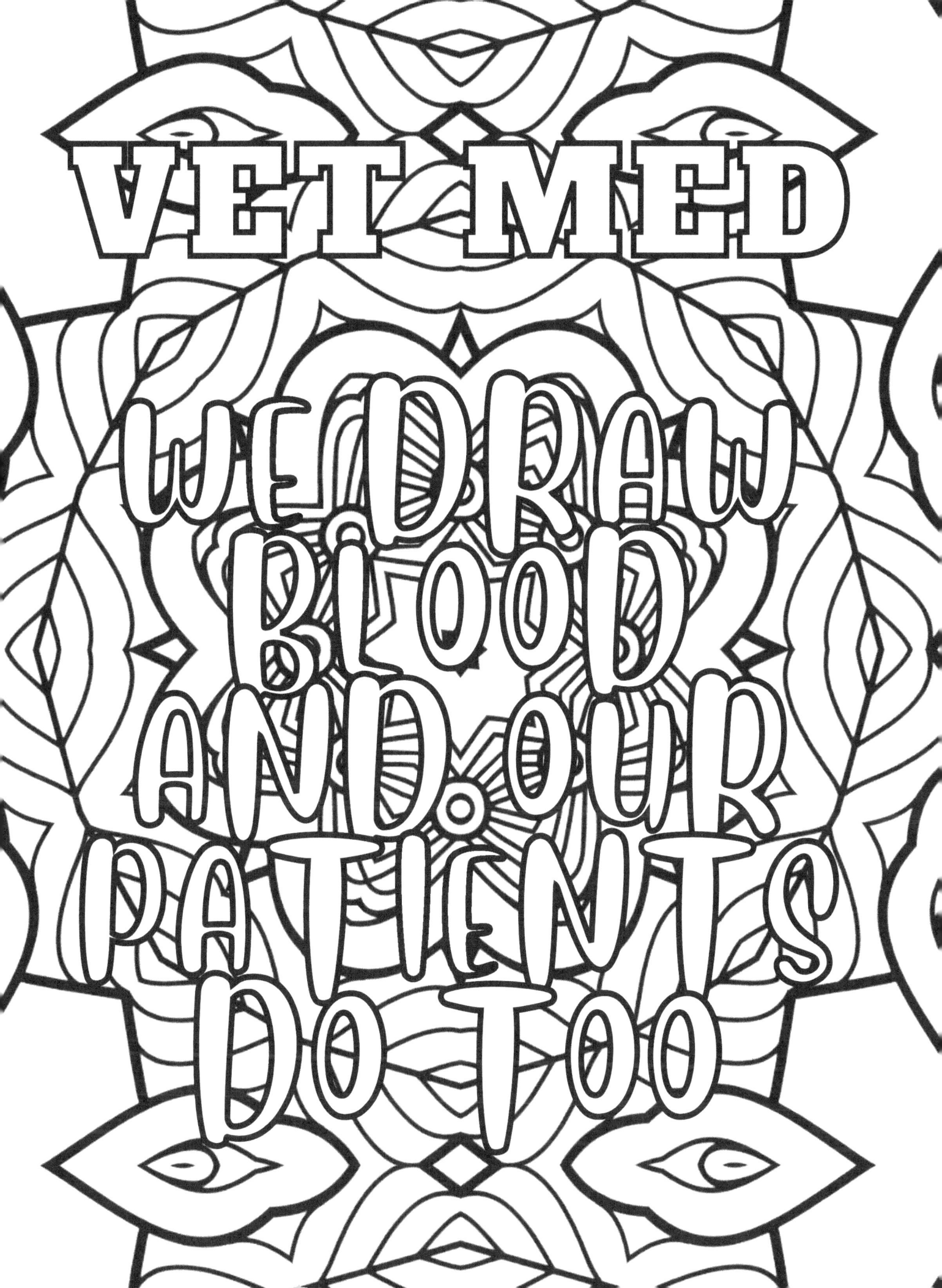

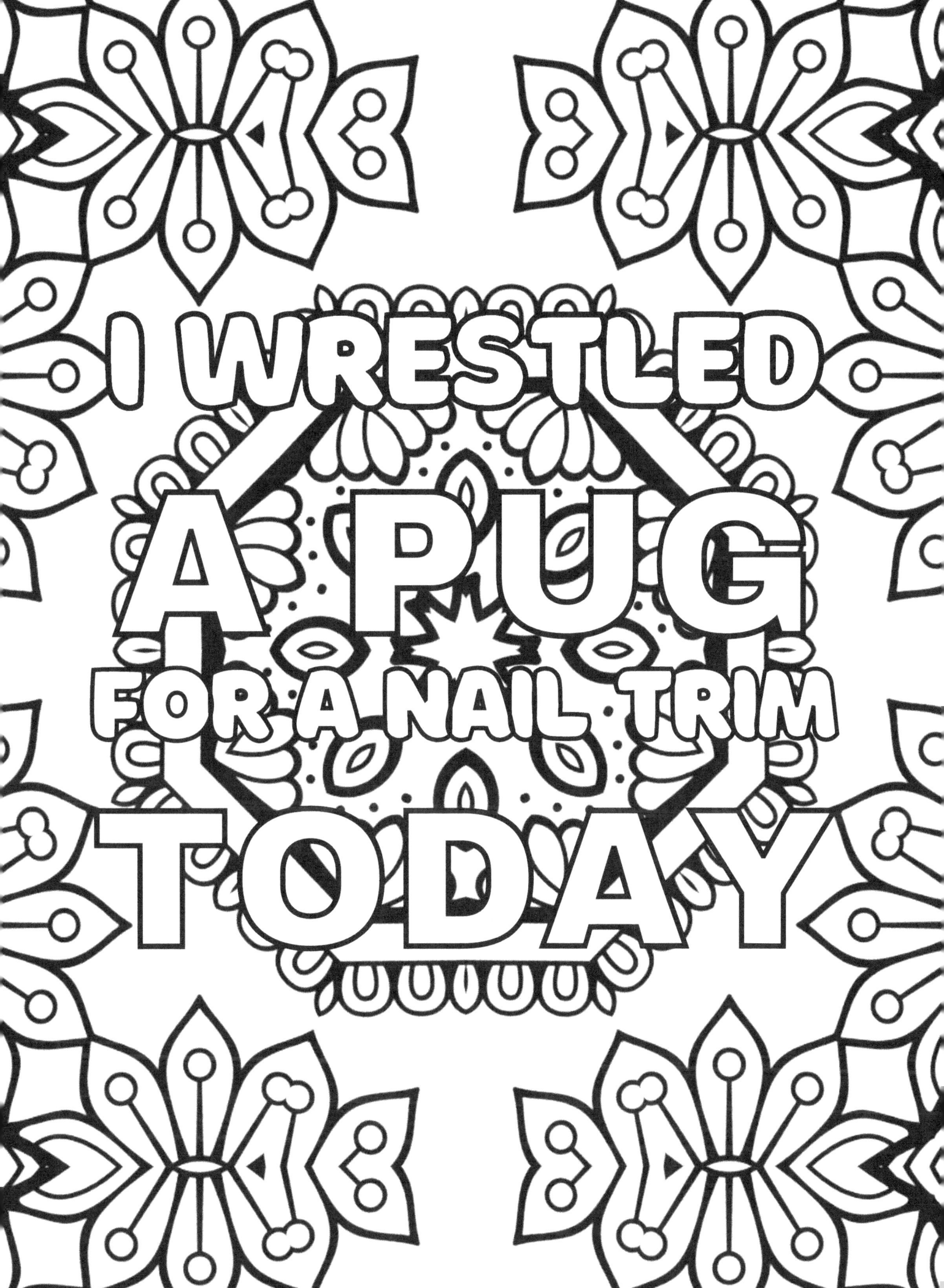

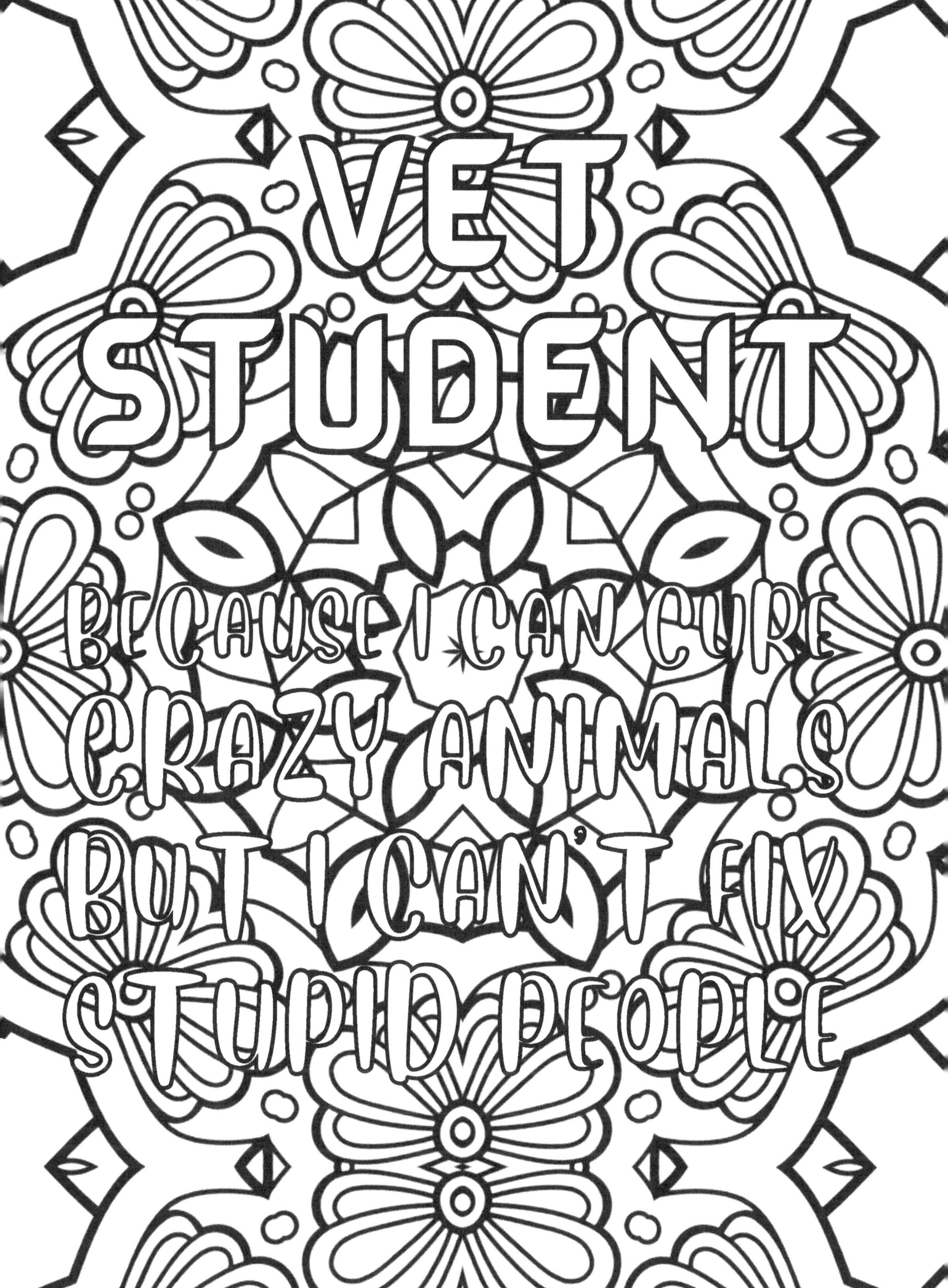

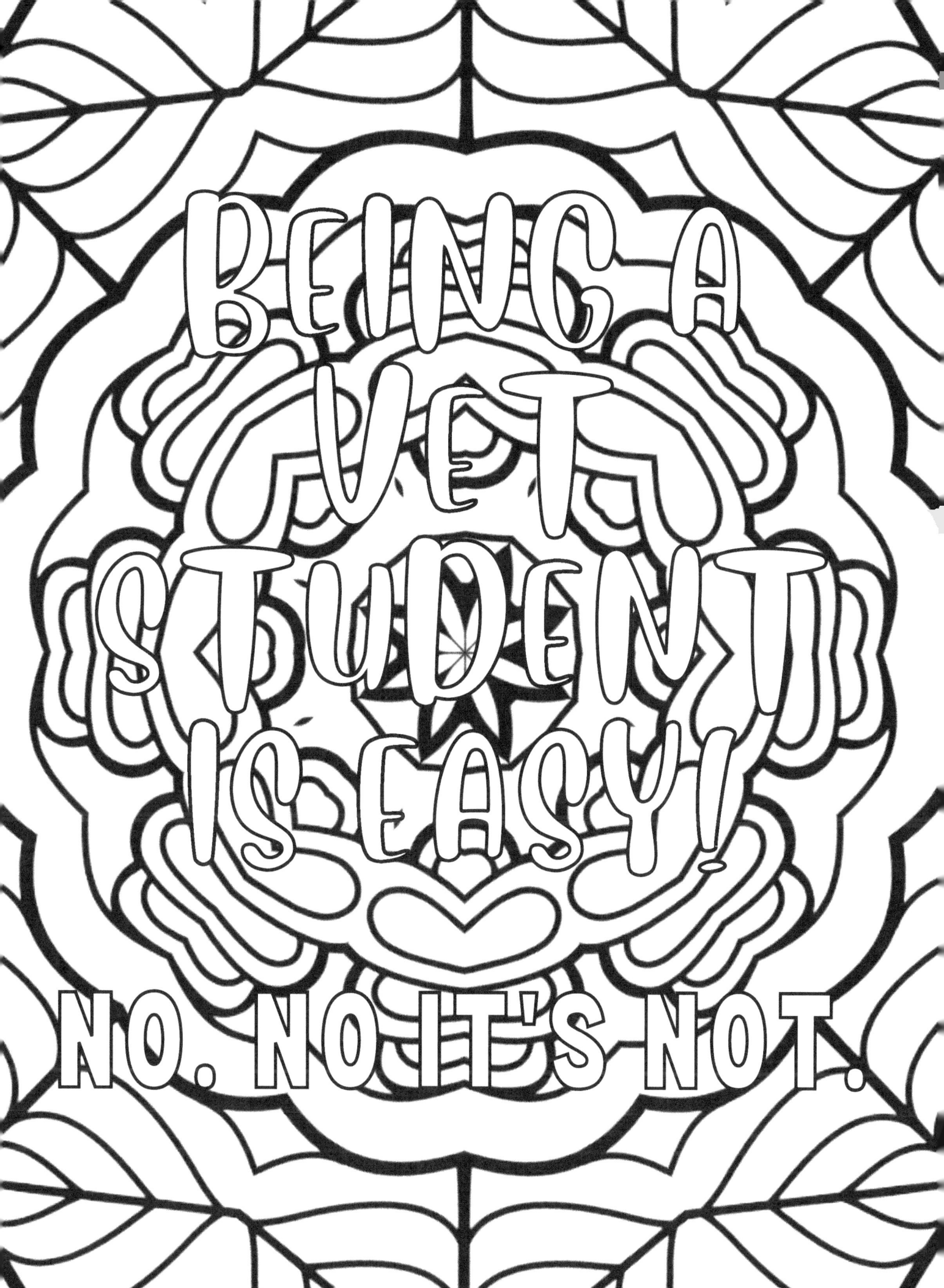

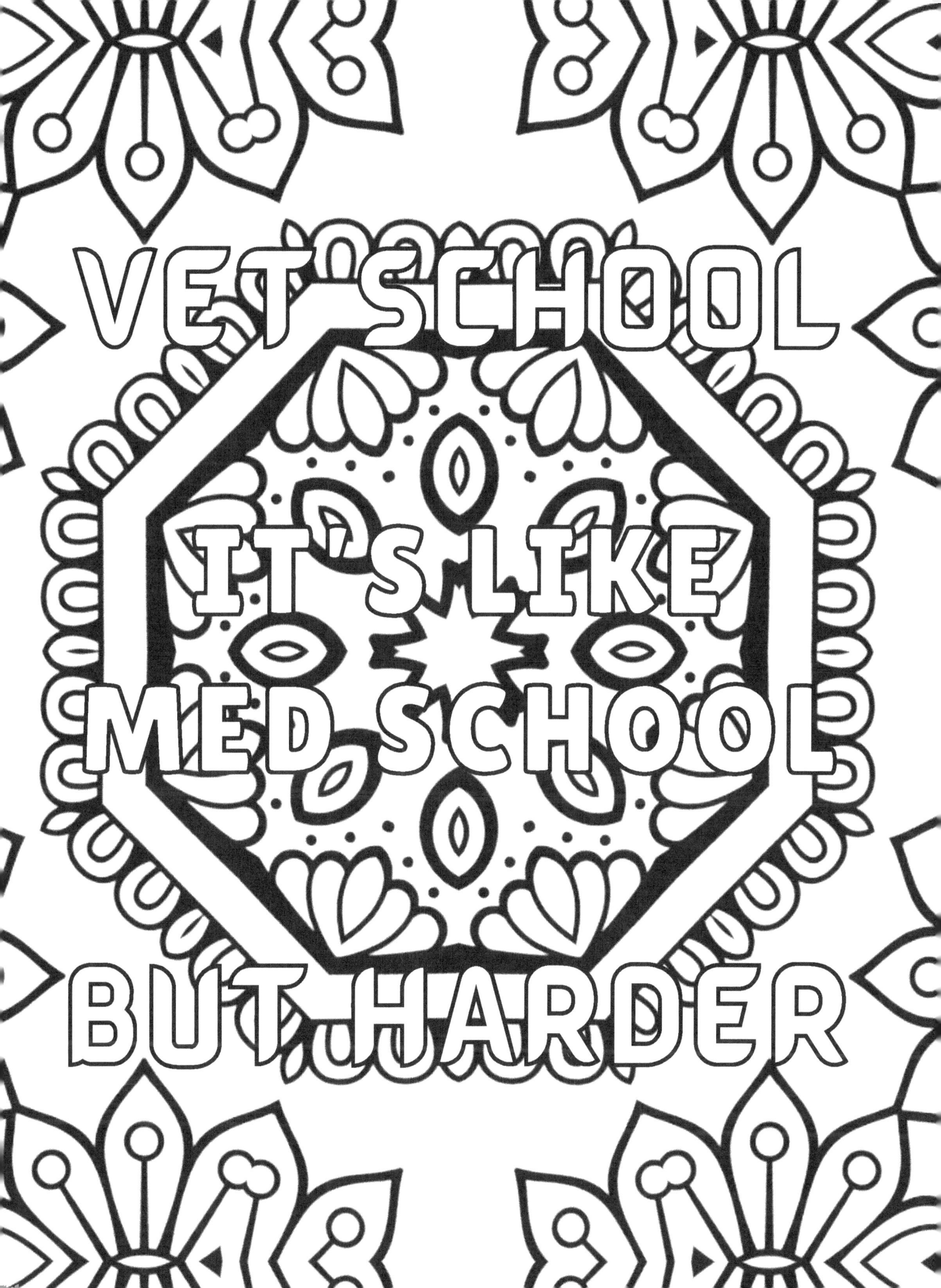

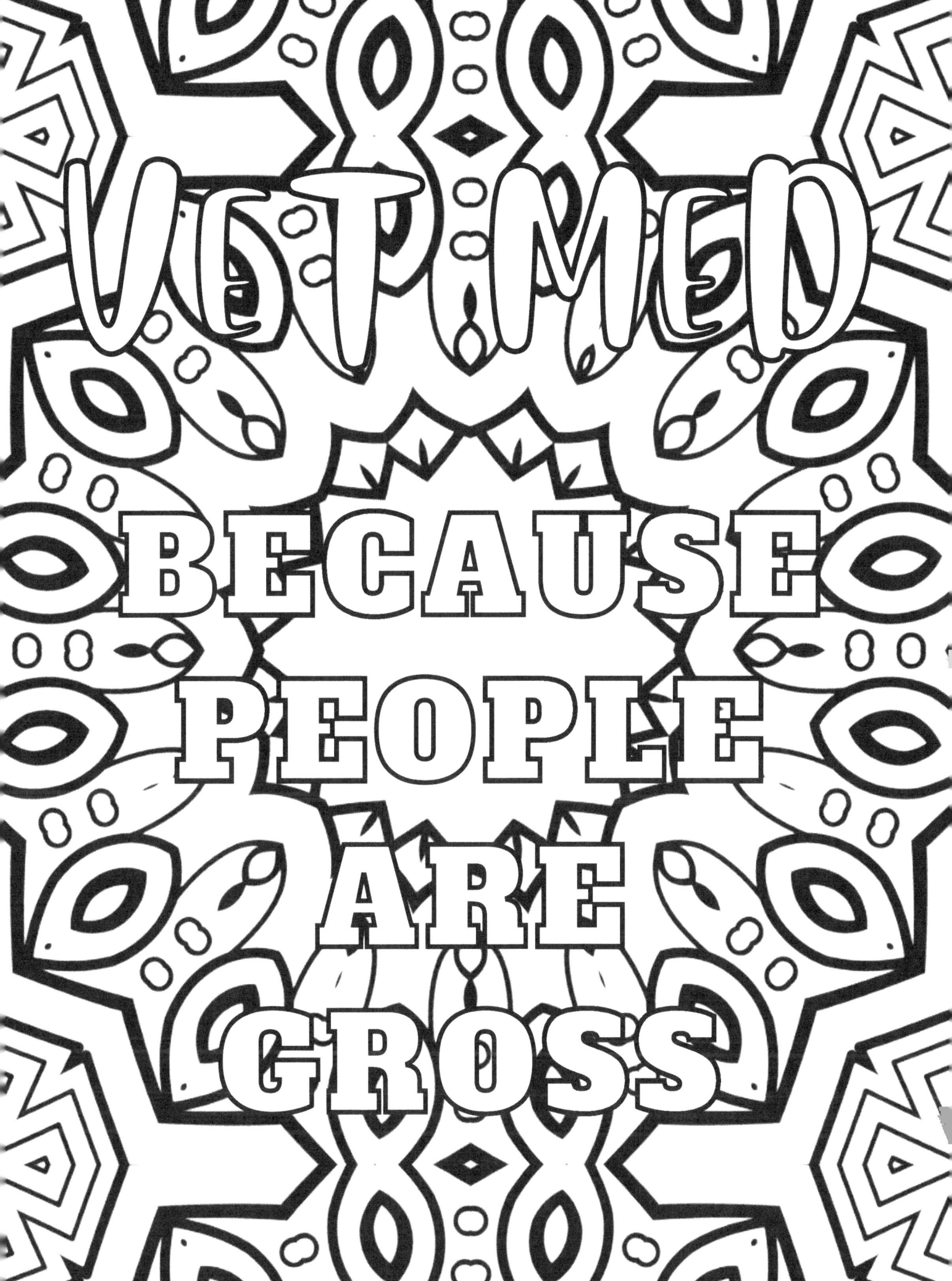

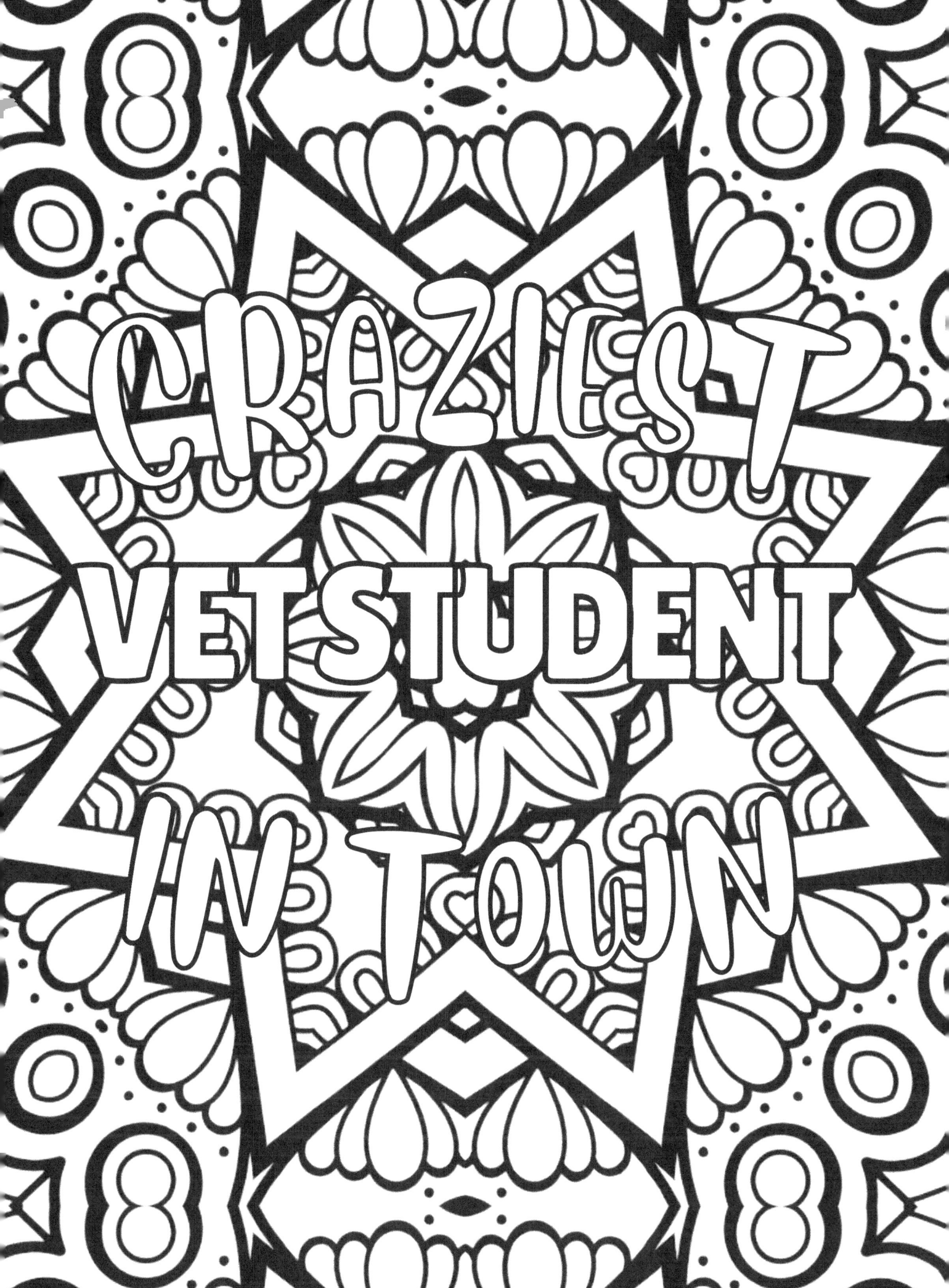

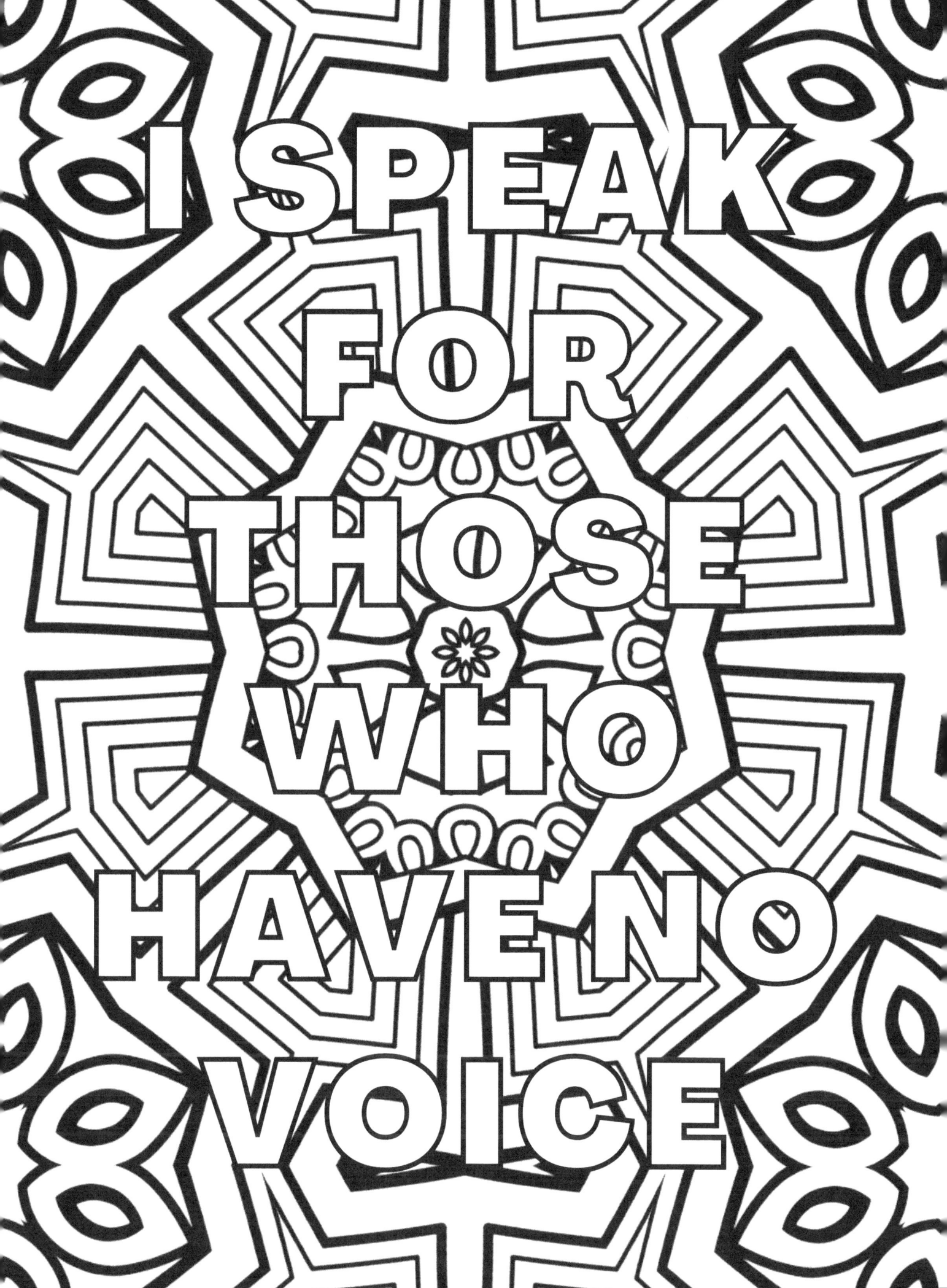

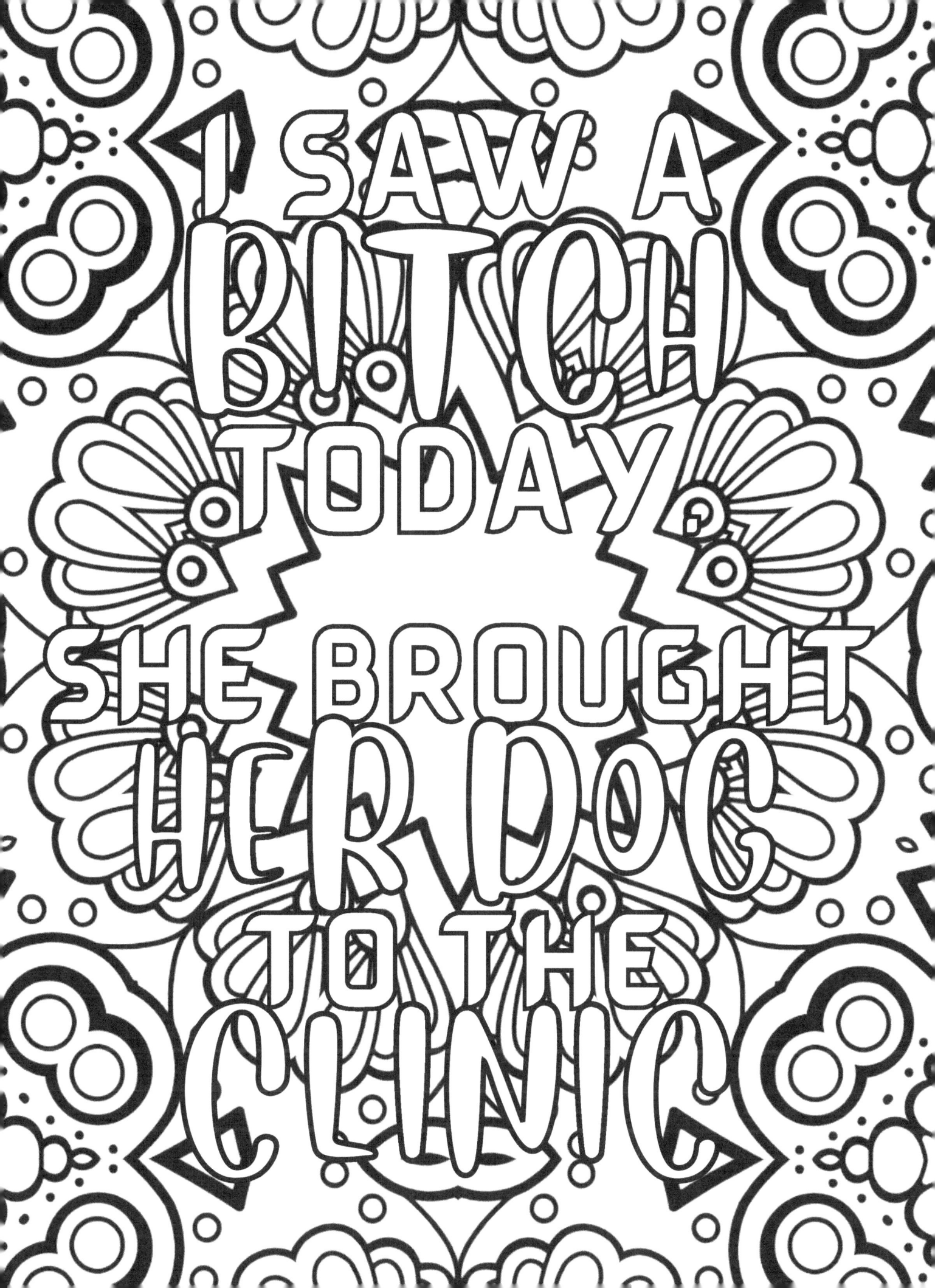

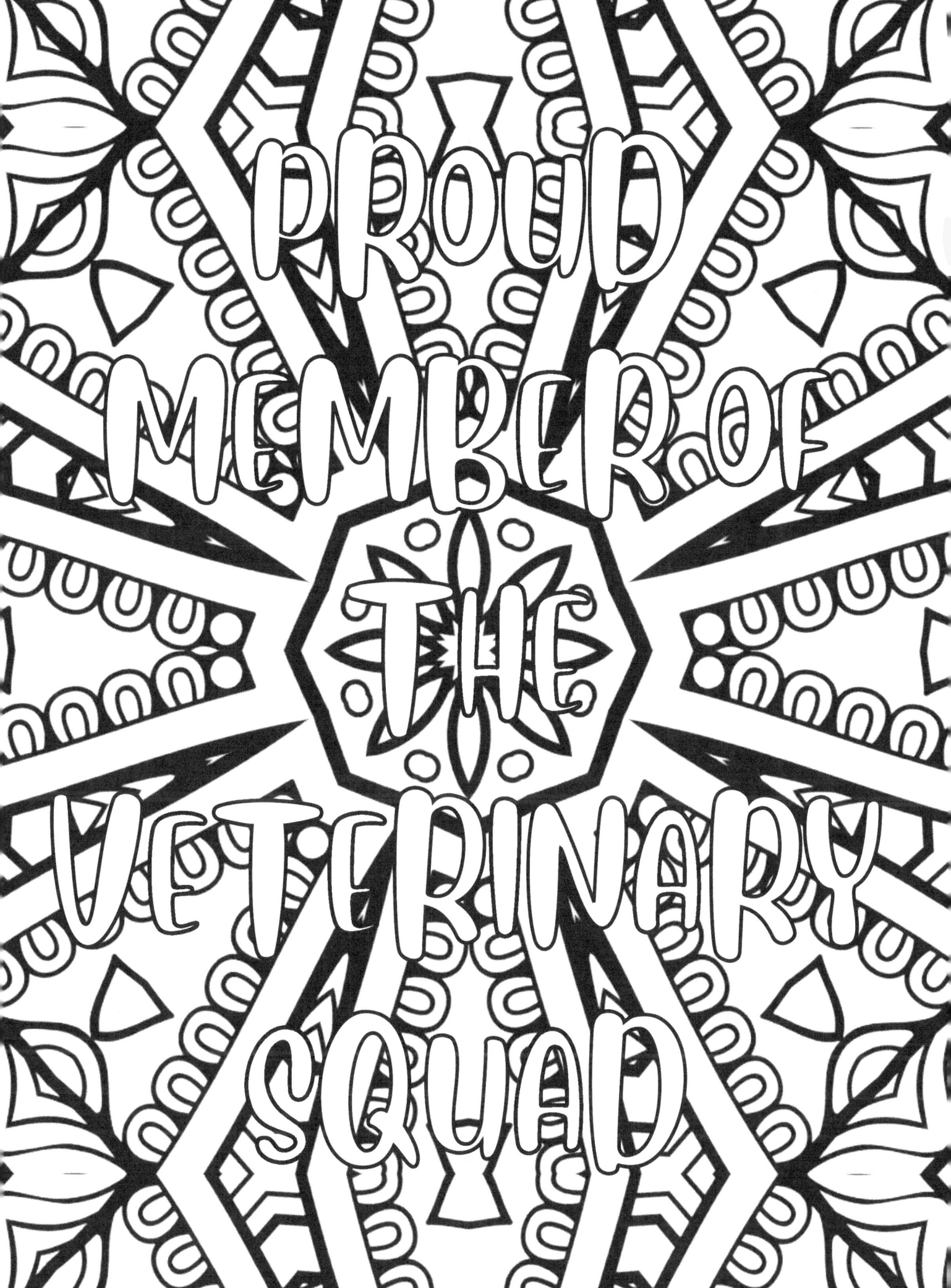

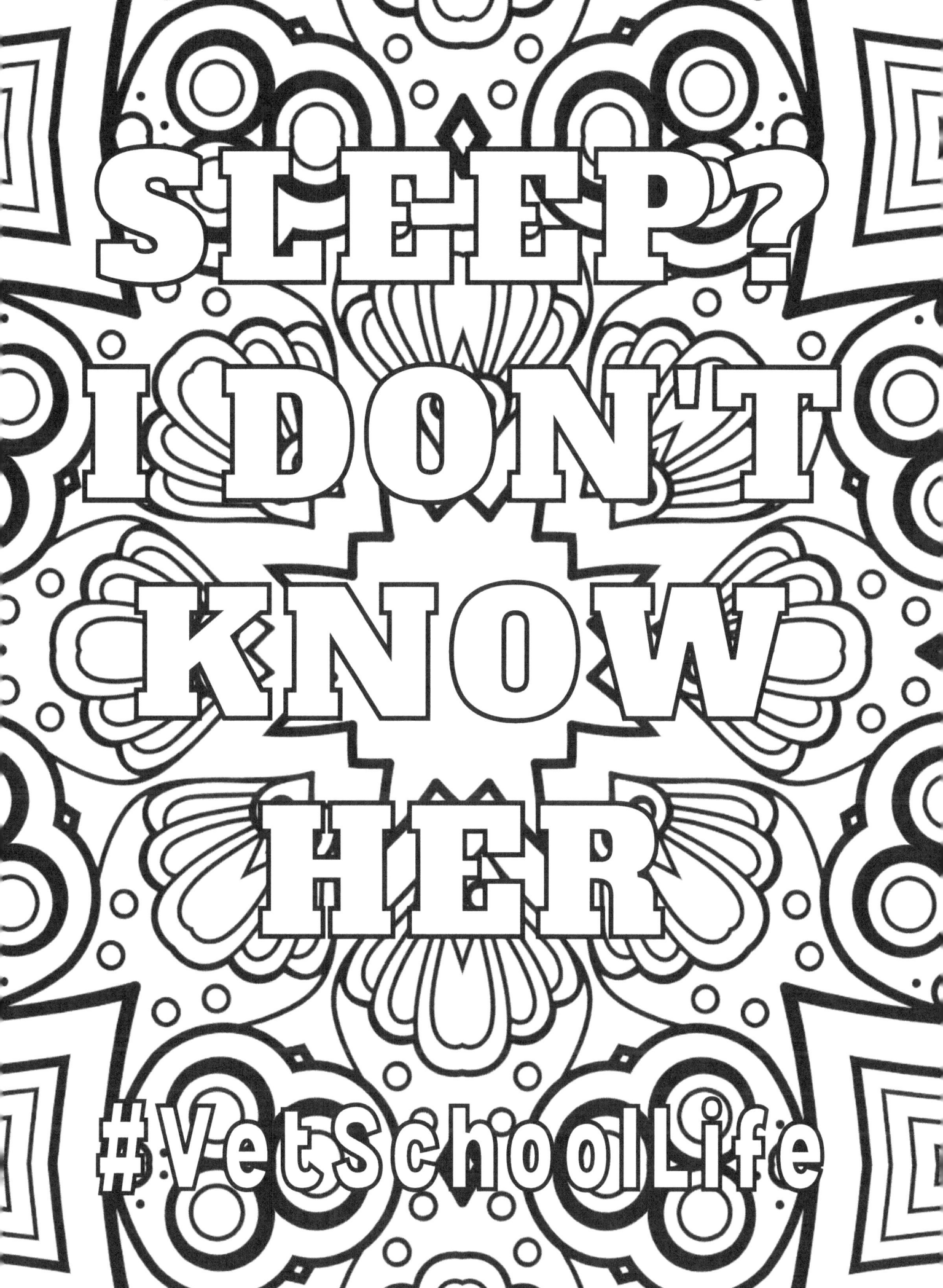

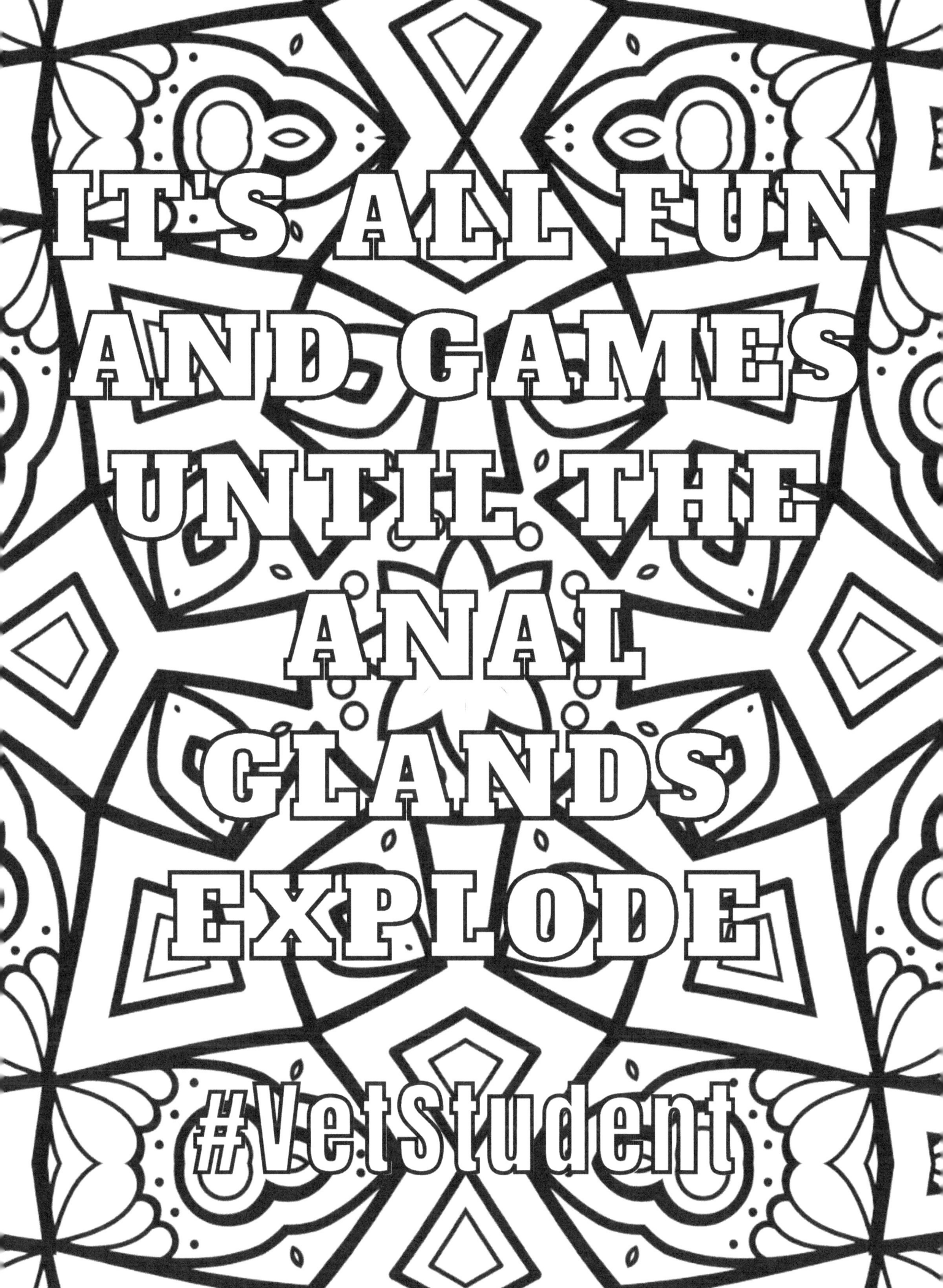

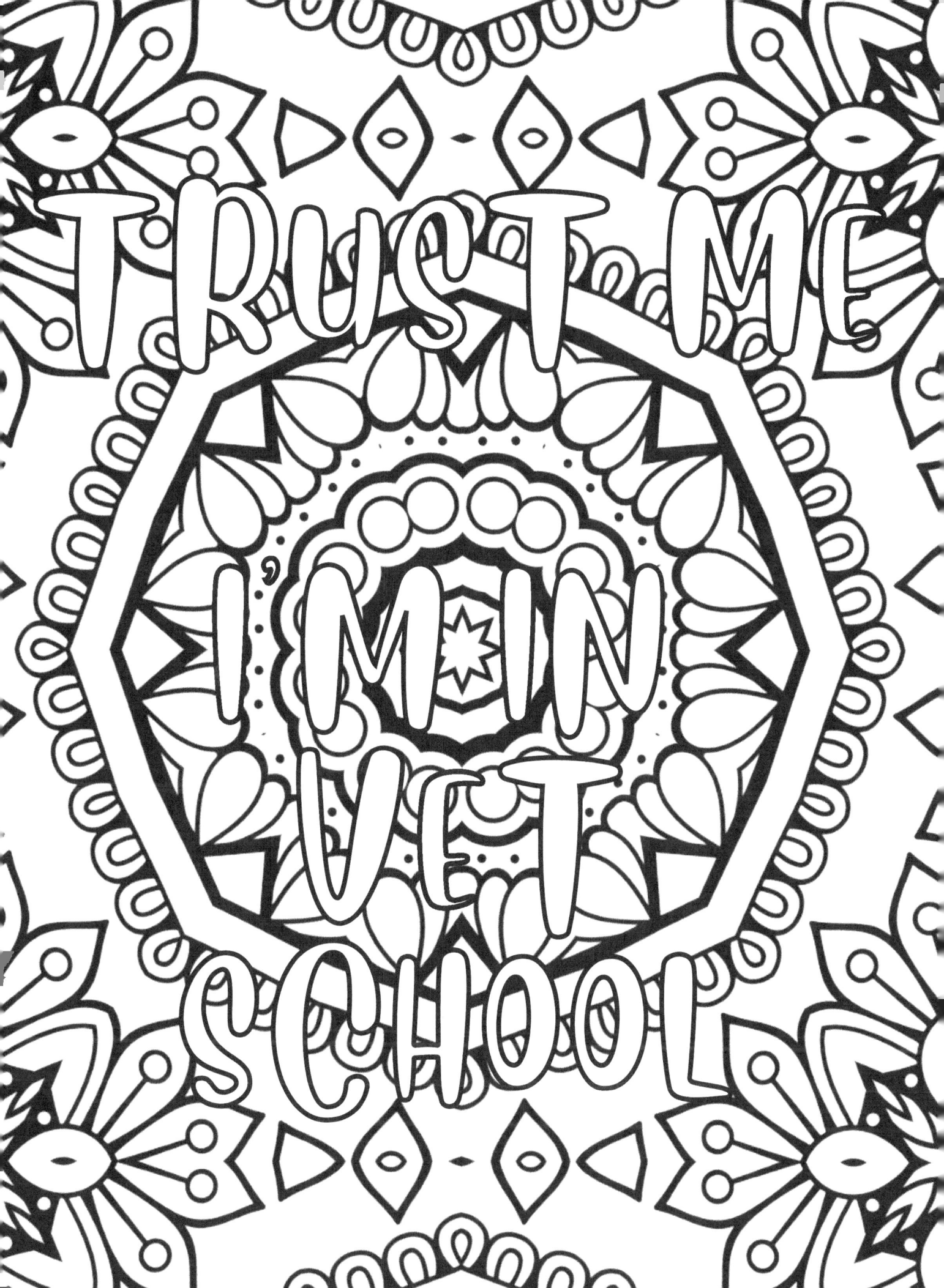

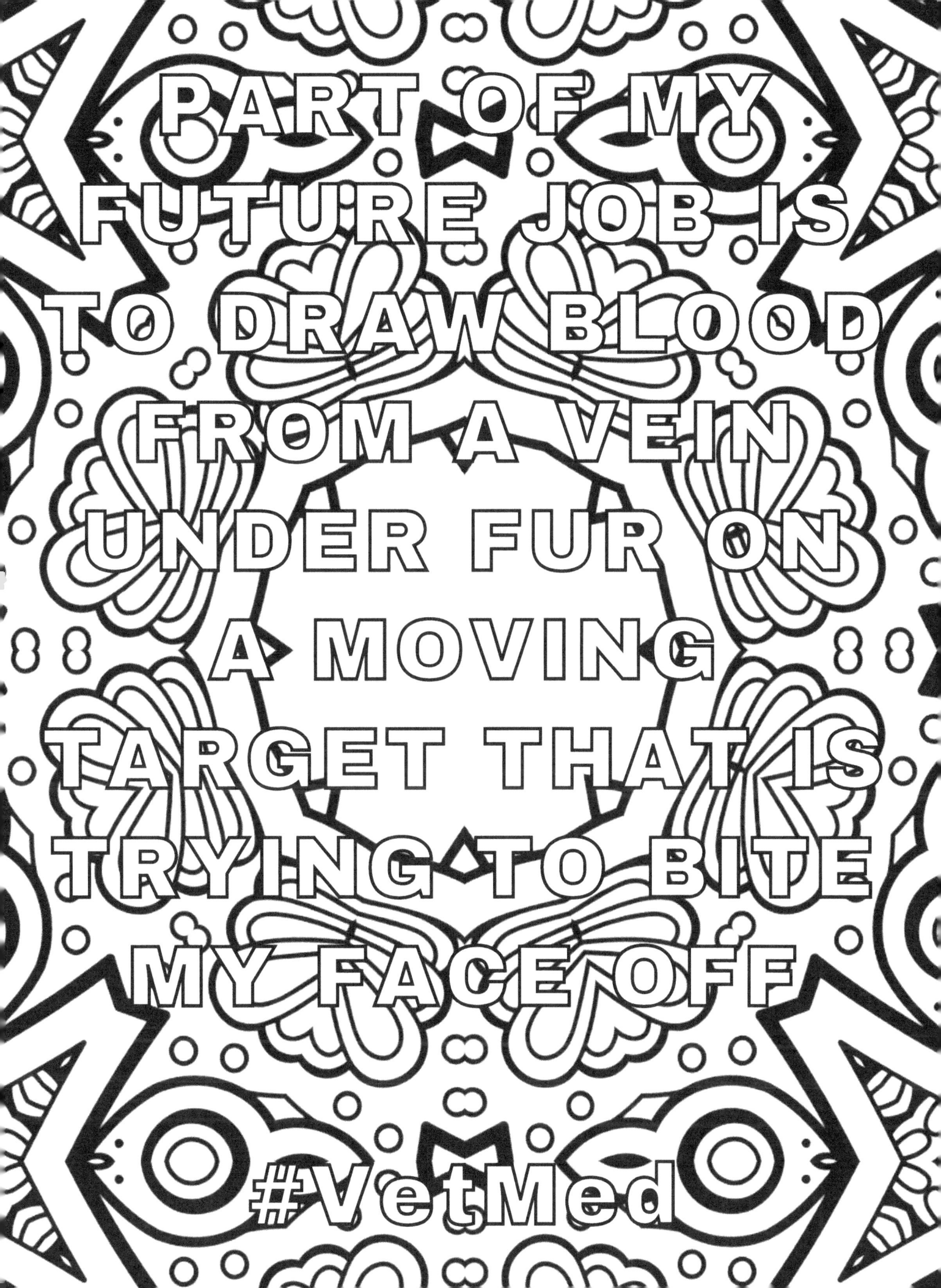

PART OF MY FUTURE JOB IS TO DRAW BLOOD FROM A VEIN UNDER FUR ON A MOVING TARGET THAT IS TRYING TO BITE MY FACE OFF

#VetMed

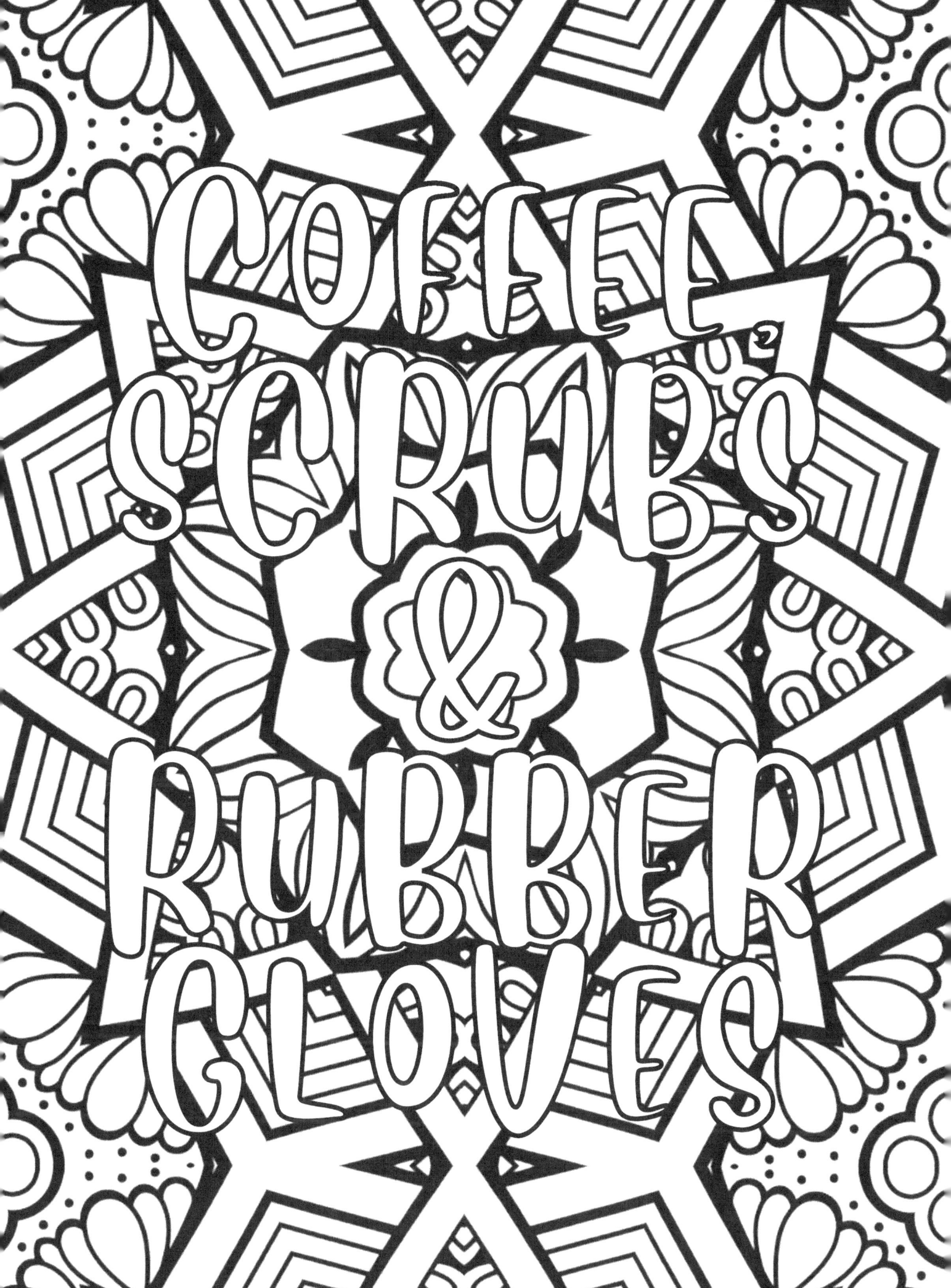

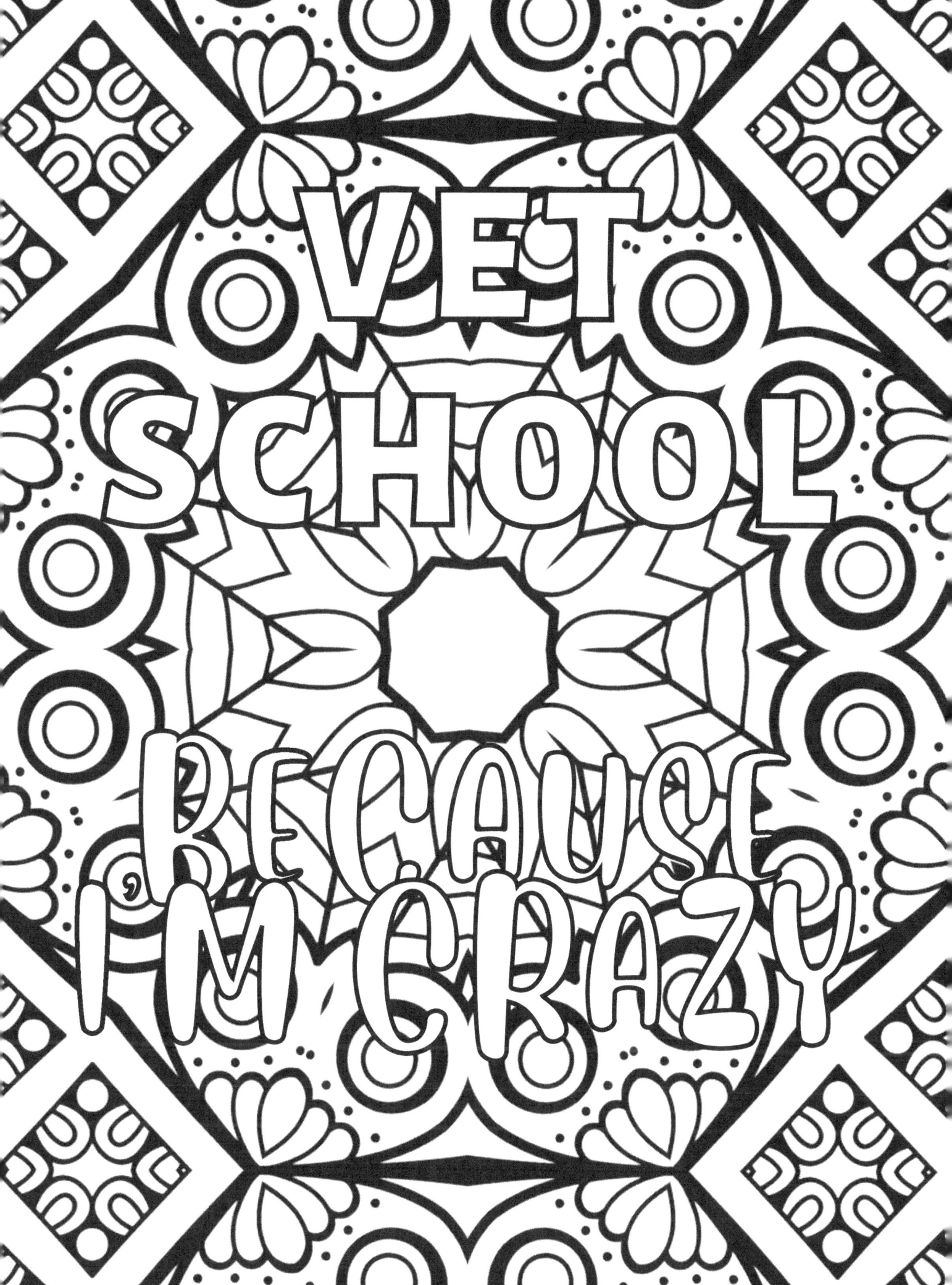

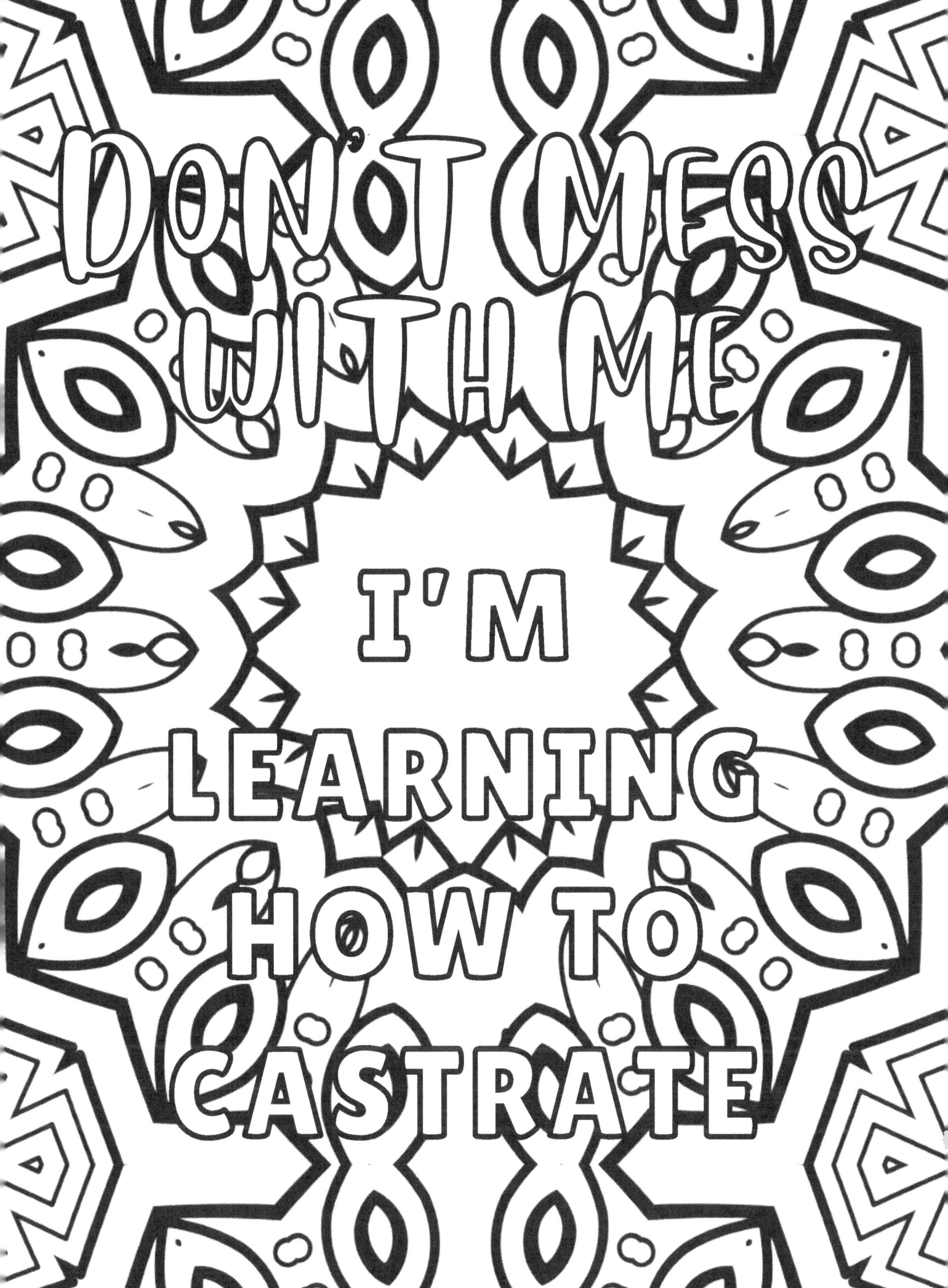

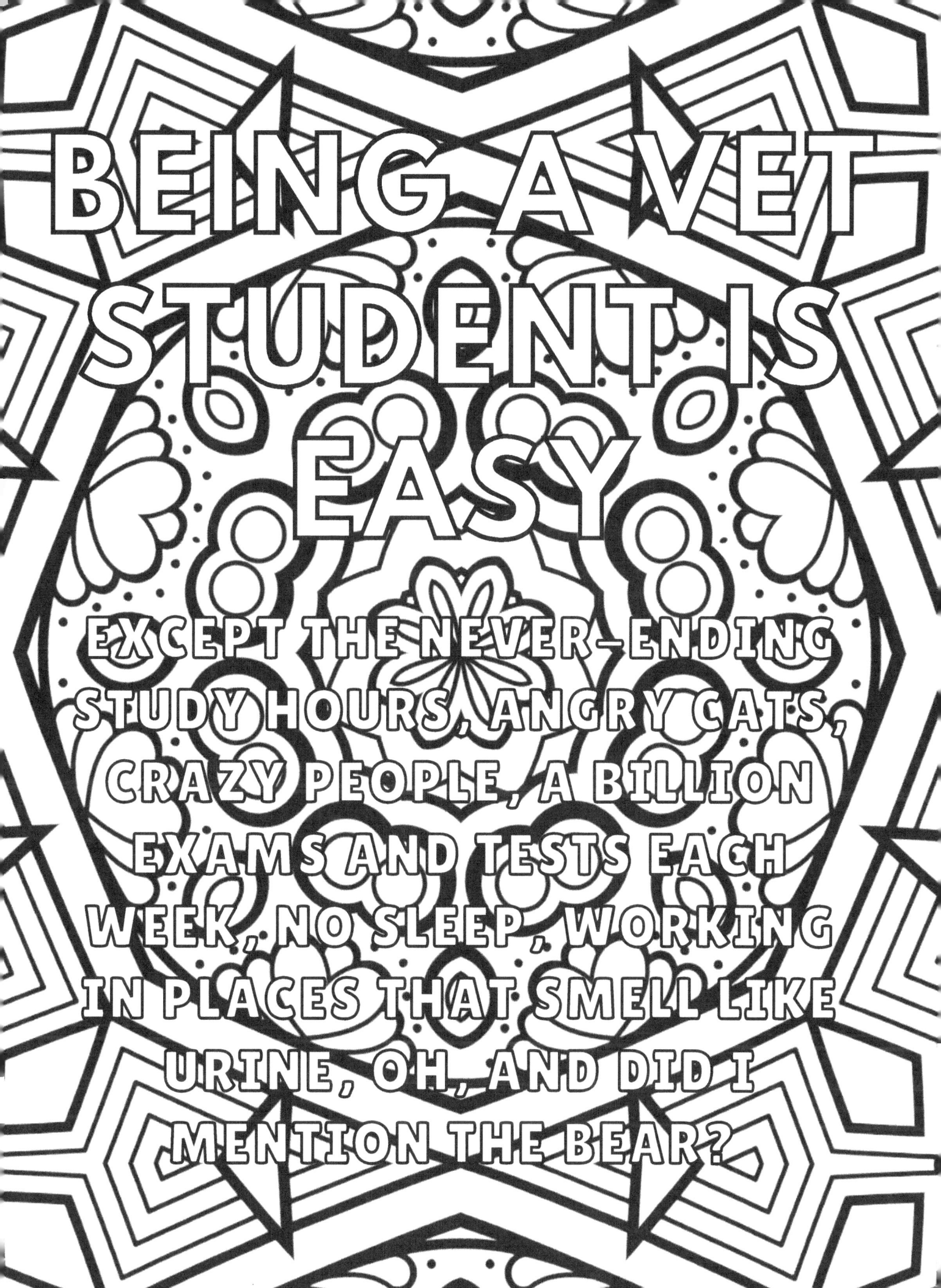